Insulin Resistance: Your Concise Guide to Preventing Diabetes

By

Reagan Prescott

Copyright © 2016

Table of Contents

1.
Introduction

Insulin is a hormone. The body produces insulin to help it regulate the body's metabolism.

The body needs energy to function, and so how the body manages this is critical. Imagine a car that could not convert gas into energy correctly. The car would soon start to stall and so it is with your body. We need to be able to convert carbohydrates, sugars and starch into glucose. This is because glucose provides us with the much-needed energy to be able to carry out normal activities. The glucose – which itself is a form of sugar – is then released into the bloodstream and this is where insulin jumps into action.

Insulin helps the cells in your body to absorb glucose at the correct level and speed. When we eat, the amount of glucose in our blood rises and glandular organ in our body called the pancreas – located just behind your stomach – releases insulin to meet up with it, and together the insulin and glucose work to ensure the correct levels of glucose are distributed throughout all the areas of your body, providing the much-needed energy produced glucose.

This as a process is finely balanced by the body and some parts of the body need the amount of glucose lowered in the bloodstream that feeds them and other parts of the body - for example, the liver - can even store glucose - this stored form of glucose is called glycogen. Once again, it is insulin that helps the liver store much-needed glucose, because it is the insulin in the bloodstream that stimulates the liver to do so.

When this does not occur, or when the insulin in our bodies is not functioning correctly, the amount of glucose that travels through the bloodstream can become overloaded, distributing too much glucose to parts of the body, causing the body to dysfunction.

When the body does not use insulin in a way that is effective, or it is dysfunctional as it releases insulin, it produces a condition called 'Insulin resistance.'

Insulin resistance is when the amount of glucose in the bloodstream becomes overloaded. The body is becoming ineffective in the regulation of insulin.

It is possible to suffer from insulin resistance for many years before you become aware that it is a serious problem. The good news is that we can take preventative measures to lessen the chances of this condition.

If we fail to take precautions, ignoring the dangers of insulin resistance, it can lead to the development of a condition known as 'Type 2 diabetes,' sometimes called 'prediabetes.' Moreover, there are some other life-long and life-changing conditions that can also be developed by insulin resistance, and this book will deal with some of these and how to take precautions against the threat of them.

In the following chapters, we will cover exactly what you need to know, to prevent diabetes from developing.

2.
The Main Causes of Insulin Resistance

Obesity

Many people think that to be classed as 'obese' one has to be very large indeed. It is now widely believed that even with a moderate excess of fat, building up, especially around the tummy area or waist, can lead to significant health problems developing.

It is now understood that excess weight is not solely a matter of amassing extra energy surpluses in the form of fatty tissue. The fat stored in the 'belly' area of the body also produces its unique set of hormones that, over time and release into the bloodstream, can lead to significant long-term health problems.

Health concerns, due to obesity, probably more widely known about can include:

High Cholesterol.

Coronary heart disease.

Some forms of Cancer [Colon, breast, gallbladder].

Stroke.

High Blood pressure.

Osteoarthritis.

It is important to note the myriad of problems, including those listed above that obesity could induce as it gives us some indication of how much stress the body can come under if it is allowed to become obese. This list is by no means exhaustive, and the primary focus of this book is to look at the condition known as insulin resistance.

When the body is put under strain, by being allowed to become obese, it causes inflammation to build up within the body, this, in turn, causes the body to react, sending immunity cells to the area of the body under duress.

When triggered, the action of immune cells on the inflamed areas of the body can cause a condition to develop called, Chronic Inflammation. Although this is termed, low-level Chronic Inflammation, it can cause the body to develop insulin resistance further. It is insulin resistance that leads to Type 2 Diabetes.

Once Type 2 Diabetes is developed within the body, the condition is now deemed to be severe indeed.

Most people that develop Type 2 Diabetes are overweight, or obese, especially around their tummy area. If you are in any doubt about whether you are in danger, you can check this out with your GP; however, a simple shirt-off glance at yourself in the mirror, will soon reveal if you would objectively consider your mid-riff as being more of a pear shape, indicating the tummy area contains more fatty deposits than is healthy, or you may be fortunate and possess a nice trim tummy area.

Losing access weight will certainly help reduce the risk of developing insulin resistance.

Lack of exercise

We cannot look into obesity problems without considering one of the main reasons why obesity can become a problem to us.

It is all to do with your muscles.

The muscles in your body use up more glucose than any other part of you. They need the energy glucose supplies to be able to function powerfully and as the glucose in their reserves gets used up, it is replaced by more and more, that is drawn out of your bloodstream. This partnership between insulin that helps control the levels of glucose in the blood and your muscles is an essential function, enabling you to keep the right amount of energy supply going into tired muscles.

The partnership between the muscles and insulin further causes the muscles to be highly sensitive to the action of insulin and can even reverse the effects of insulin resistance, which in turn causes the glucose levels in the bloodstream to lower when they become too high.

This action in the body demonstrates the essential nature of taking regular exercise and how important it is to keep those muscles working.

The more that the muscles are developed in the body means, the more they can burn off excess glucose being supplied to them. This ensures that glucose levels are not in danger of becoming and being maintained at a level that is too high, or that may become hazardous for the body.

So you can see that if one does not take regular exercise, the risk of glucose levels becoming too high is very real and as such is not a very good idea, as it is putting the body in a risky situation.

We start to see a vicious circle of body activity as we look at the causes of insulin resistance, as the likelihood of someone becoming dangerously overweight is much higher if they take little or no exercise at all.

A person, who is overweight and can testify to not exercising, stands a greater chance of developing insulin resistance than one who is conscious of taking daily exercise, while keeping an eye on that expanding waistline.

Poor sleep patterns

Sleep is an essential part of our lives, as you would find if you tried to stay awake and alert, even through the duration of just one single night.

The body takes a time-out while we are asleep, repairing and resting the areas that need maintenance. The body enjoys a mini-service each night if you like.

One particular problem related to sleep that can be particularly relevant as we look at the causes of insulin resistance is one called sleep apnea. Sleep apnea is when the patterns of our sleep are disrupted. This means that we do not get a good night sleep even if we believe we have because we have been asleep all night.

Sleep apnea causes the levels of carbon dioxide in the bloodstream to increase and this, in turn, signals to your body that it is time to wake up. One can experience many episodes of sleep apnea during one session of sleep, and this means that you are in and out of deep sleep, rather than enjoying a consecutive session of relaxing, repairing, and continuous, deep sleep.

The problem with sleep apnea is that it causes one to go into a shallow breathing state, from a deep sleep state during sleep, and this causes the quality of the sleep you are experiencing to be reduced. This, in turn, causes an individual to feel tired and listless during the day, experiencing reduced energy levels.

This condition is linked to high levels of obesity and insulin resistance, leading to Type 2 Diabetes, if you think about it, who wants to think about taking exercise when their sleep has made them tired enough?

As this link is quite strong, it is important that you seek help from your health provider if you think you suffer from sleep apnea. The common symptoms are:

Waking sleep during the day. This is a daydreaming state that causes one to feel otherworldly, or as if they are drifting off continually during daily routines.

Excessive snoring can be a sign that the body is not enjoying the sleep it needs.

Extreme tiredness, leading to difficulties concentrating and sometimes blurred vision.

Other dangers

Ethnicity

This is an interesting one and has more to do with evolution and the movement of people groups than having a poor health regime.

Human beings have evolved over hundreds and thousands of years, and so, human blood glucose levels have evolved along with every other part of our body.

Insulin sensitivity and insulin response are two variables of a term within the bodies functioning systems called, hyperbolic function. This delicate balance arrangement within our bodies has regulated hyperbolic function to suit the environment we live in.

However, humans have a huge capacity to move around or migrate. As we move around the globe, we can sometimes find ourselves pushed to the furthermost spectrum of our particular area of population stability – this stability feature is called canalization. It is now believed that differences can now be found within the optimal states of both insulin sensitivity and what we are looking at, which is insulin resistance.

One recent study, Khan et al., (2013) looked at the likelihood of three people groups, namely Caucasians, Africans and East Asians, being more or less susceptible to the most unstable end of the spectrum that we are discussing here.

If you imagine a straight line running from A-B and believe this line is a spectrum - or range of possible outcomes - results suggested in this study that Caucasians were more in the middle of the line between A-B and risk of imbalance regarding their body being vulnerable to insulin sensitivity and insulin resistance. The metabolisms of Africans and East Asians were shown as being pushed more toward the extreme ends of the spectrum, thus indicating a possible link toward a higher propensity to this condition.

Therefore, again, it is worth checking out the possibility of ethnically related vulnerability toward insulin resistance, as this may warrant a little more execution of preventative measures.

Old age

Admittedly, there is nothing we can do to halt time and as our bodies start to deteriorate, getting less exercise, with all the temptations to indulge ourselves with a little bit of what we fancy, we are more susceptible to most health problems. Therefore, it is advisable to get checked out regularly, ensuring your diet is as good as it can be and that you are taking as many precautions as you can to hold of the consequences of time.

Cigarette smoking

Chemicals found in cigarettes do react unfavorably with glucose levels in the body, and so if you have been, or you still are quite a heavy smoker, it is advisable once again to check out how you might best lower the chances of becoming more vulnerable to insulin resistance. Of course giving up smoking is always going to be beneficial to one's health and if that thought is intolerable to you, at least think seriously about cutting down.

Use of steroids

The use of steroids [full name Corticosteroids] is quite widespread, usually to reduce inflammation and suppress the immune system.

A GP may prescribe steroids if you have acute asthma, or if there is constant, isolated inflammation occurring in your body due to conditions such as arthritis.

Prednisone is the name of a commonly used steroid. This steroid can interfere with the glucose levels in your body, causing those levels to rise significantly.

As with any drug, hormone, or another chemical, introduced to the bloodstream, affecting the levels of glucose, it is wise to recognize that this particular steroid can increase the possibility of insulin resistance

3.
Prediabetes

What is Prediabetes?

It is important to know what prediabetes is if we are going to be fully equipped to do all we can to avoid being diagnosed with diabetes.

Prediabetes could also be described as borderline diabetes and as the pre, before diabetes indicates, it is not actual Type 2 diabetes, but a prelude condition, we need to be aware of.

Prediabetes is when the blood glucose levels are high and could be in danger of rising even higher or causing Type 2 diabetes. The levels of glucose are elevated, but not high enough for a Type 2 diabetes diagnosis.

People who suffer from insulin resistance are more prone to suffer from prediabetes. However, insulin resistance does not necessarily lead to Type 2 diabetes.

It is important to note that even if you do suffer from prediabetes, this does not necessarily mean you are certain to contract Type 2 diabetes. High and rising levels of glucose concentrations in the blood put pressure on the body to deal with it efficiently and impair your ability to distribute the glucose in the bloodstream efficiently. Prediabetes may well be the warning someone might need to take action now, avoiding the ever-rising possibilities that they are vulnerable to Type 2 diabetes.

Blood glucose levels & ranges

Knowing more about blood glucose levels and ranges should prompt us in our understanding, that the process of calculating correct levels and ranges can be quite a complicated process. Do we need to be asking ourselves if we need to consult with our health-care provider in case any adjustments in our lifestyle are required, for us to avoid contracting diabetes?

There are two main methods used to measure glucose in the bloodstream:

The chemical testing process. This approach exploits the nonspecific reducing property of glucose in the blood, using a substance as an indicator of levels of glucose reduction. When this method is used, the index material will change color if the levels are reduced. This approach can be utilized using blood, or urine as samples. The samples are exposed to the indicator chemical substance on a strip, which is then inserted into a meter to ascertain a reading, or compared to a color chart, for the same purposes. The urine sample test is still in operation today, but the blood sample test is now not used. The accuracy of these tests has come under considerable scrutiny in recent years, due to the accuracy levels being criticized. The second method [below] is preferred in the modern age.

The enzyme testing process. This uses enzymes instead of chemicals to measure the amount of glucose present. The enzymes employed are, glucose itself, oxidase and hexokinase. This method is now viewed as the one that will give a greater degree of accuracy.

It is important to note that blood sugar / glucose levels and results should always be discussed with a qualified clinician, as there can be a variation of interpretation of results of measuring these levels between different individuals.

A good understanding of the various levels and ranges of glucose concentrations in the bloodstream is the first step towards us being able to manage how high our vulnerability to diabetes may be.

It is likely that you would be asked to fast before being tested for levels of glucose in your blood, as the activity of eating food, can upset the metabolic system, causing the results to fluctuate too much to be able to give a consistent level result.

When you get your blood sugar / level tested, you will find that there are various ranges of blood glucose levels to be considered. We mentioned prediabetes above and as with all ranges, your individual level of blood glucose will be unique to you and determine whether you are suffering from prediabetes, or at risk of diabetes. For example, one reading may mean the results impact on one person, slightly differently than the same reading on another person. Medical advice is always of paramount importance when considering the interpretation of medical results.

The important thing to consider – if you think you may be in danger of contracting diabetes - is a culmination of your blood glucose results from your health care provider, whether that reading is rising and of course, your lifestyle and diet.

Some of the blood glucose ranges that can become evident, as a result of being tested for possible high blood glucose levels are:

Standard range – This is obviously where you want to be if you are in no immediate danger of contracting diabetes.

Prediabetes range – As stated above, these ranges will include results that are individually interpreted.

The range for, adults and children with Type 1. Diabetes.

The range for, adults and children with Type 2. Diabetes.

Should you be tested for prediabetes?

Some of the indicators, guiding us whether or not we need to be tested for prediabetes, or insulin resistance, can be found within the lifestyle we lead. Suffice it to say, all of us should be having regular checkups from our healthcare providers, as mentioned earlier and as we develop into older age, the necessity for these checkups become more frequent.

All symptoms that are developed in the body – if they are what you would consider abnormal to you, or new and worrying changes in how your body is functioning – should be checked out.

If you are aware that your lifestyle is not one that includes daily exercise, and you are noticing that you carry excess weight, again, the need for regular checkups and blood sugar / glucose tests are a very good idea.

One can be insulin resistant and have a body that is in a condition of prediabetes for many years and be totally unaware of it. Healthcare providers will look for indicators; that will point to the level of risk that you carry and these indicators may prompt them to test for these conditions.

The Indicators

Here are some signs that may suggest a higher possibility of insulin resistance and prediabetes:

Much has already been said about lack of exercise, but if you are a bit of a couch potato, it's not great news for your body for some different reasons, not least standing as a leader in the risks of diabetes.

As with lack of exercise, obesity is a significant predictive indicator, therefore, if you know or suspect you are overweight, you are at risk.

Diabetes does have genetic links, which is why doctors often ask you, 'does anyone in your family suffer from any major health problems?'

Ethnicity links to diabetes are relevant, and so if you are: African American, Alaska Native, American Indian, Asian American, Hispanic/Latino, or Pacific Islander American, then this is another indicator you may be in a higher risk category.

Mothers who give birth to babies that are 9lb plus.

Mothers who may have developed Gestational diabetes, which is a type of diabetes, can get during the term of their pregnancies.

You are more at risk if you have a high blood pressure.

HDL cholesterol is known as friendly cholesterol because it moves through your bloodstream removing harmful cholesterol. If you have low levels of HDL cholesterol, you are more of a risk.

Triglycerides are the fats found in meat, dairy products and some cooking oils. We need to keep our eye on these fatty enzymes because they are on the list if they are too high.

Women who suffer from PCOS, or Polycystic ovary syndrome.

If you have previously suffered from prediabetes, you need to be continually aware that you are managing the possibility of its return.

Acanthosis nigricans is the medical term that explains thickened, dark patches of skin that can develop in the armpits, groin, and neck. The condition is often linked to an underlying problem – usually cancer, or obesity diabetes.

CVD or Cardiovascular disease is another indicator that points to the high possibility of insulin resistance and / or prediabetes.

Body Mass Index [BMI]

As we start to investigate whether we believe ourselves to be overweight, or not, we need to consider Body Mass Index measurements.

Body image can be a misleading and very subjective process. As we look at ourselves in the mirror, it is often easier to see a picture of what we think we should look like, or be repelled if we do not look the way we believe we ought.

If we do not look the way we think, or the way glossy magazines have often been accused of portraying how we should look, it may be easy to fall into the trap of thinking we are obese, when indeed we are not.

A useful tool that measures the mass weight of an individual against the height they stand at.

It is of little value to think of someone who is very heavy, as being obese, as his or her height may well compensate for the accrued weight carried. The reason why it is important to conduct tests such as the BMI test is to put to bed a lot of assumptions as to whether we are overweight or not. The same could be said of course for being underweight. People who are carrying little excess weight are not always the healthiest among us, and one can be underweight due to health problems, just as easily as carrying excess weight can be alarming to our risk to illnesses.

The BMI of an individual is determined by measuring and consequently plotting on a graph – Index - the mass weight of our body, divided by the square calculation of our height. The results are measured in units of kg/m2. Therefore, the measurement is the weight mass in kilograms, divided by the square of the body height.

The reason why a BMI test may be useful is that it will indicate the amount of total tissue mass, made up of muscle, fat, and bone. Essentially it measures whether or not one is over / under weight compared with how tall they are.

It should be obvious that this is a very useful measurement when we come to a decision whether we are obese, or not and it answers questions about our general level of fitness, that in turn help us to discover whether we are at risk of carrying too much fatty tissue, causing us to become vulnerable to insulin resistance and diabetes.

4.
What Can We Do to Lessen the Risk of Diabetes?

While you cannot prevent Type 1 diabetes, it is believed that nearly 60% of Type 2 diabetes can be either delayed or avoided altogether. You may be unfortunate insomuch as, you may have inherited genes that are more susceptible to contracting Type 2 diabetes, but mainly, it is lifestyle that will determine your fate.

So, what can you and I do to reduce the risks?

Eating sensibly

Some of us never like to hear it, but the fuel we fill our body with can often determine the manner in which they function.

This is particularly the case as the years go by and the cumulative effect of many years eating the wrong foods consistently can ultimately catch up with us.

The good news is that it is never too late to change our habits.

The word 'diet' often fills us with thoughts of starvation, missing out on treats and having a miserable time. Avoiding Type 2 diabetes is more about the choices we make, rather than the amount of food we consume.

Eating what dieticians call a balanced diet is critical, as all the food groups needed to sustain a healthy mind and body need to be taken into our bodies, ensuring all of the bodily functions are catered for.

Eating a balanced diet will not only boost our immunity system, but it will also cause us to feel better generally, feel more alert and stop us becoming tired too easily.

Food is readily available to most people living in the Western world and over the years the size or portion of our meals have grown, as we take advantage of the choice of food available to us.

A good first step to eating more healthy meals is to cut down on the size of your meals. This will result in your body expecting less, over time and reduce the amount of excess food sugars stored up and maintained within the body in the form of fatty tissue.

Try and compliment your meals with a good healthy supply of fruit and vegetables, as they are rich in vitamins and minerals and low in fats and calories.

Some golden rules to remember as you strive to maintain a healthy diet are:

Try and eat five pieces of fruit and veg a day.

Pick starchy foods that contain more fiber. So rather than continually reaching for the old favorites such as potatoes, rice, and bread – as they contain carbohydrates, that are turned into glucose by your body - try reaching further, for fiber rich, starchy food, such as, wholegrain bread, wholegrain pasta and basmati.

Fresh food will always contain more vitamins and minerals than processed food.

Low-fat foods will always contain less fat than full-fat foods.

Your healthcare provider can offer much more advice regarding healthy eating and if you need a lot of help, ask to be referred to a dietician.

Exercising properly

Diet and exercise are the most important and efficient ways to ward off the threat of diabetes and as we learned earlier, if our muscles are working, they are burning off excess glucose, reducing the risk of building it up in the body, which in turn heightens the risk of developing diabetes.

It is thought that up to 40% of patients suffering from diabetes could have avoided the condition, solely by exercising regularly.

Exercising regularly is also believed to aid people once they have been unfortunate enough to contract Type 2 diabetes, as patients have repeatedly testified to cutting down on the amount of insulin they need to take in, once the benefits of exercising have kicked in.

As with all activities that are introduced into your daily routine - especially if one is not already in good physical condition – one should seek medical advice, as excessive strain on a body that is not used to it can prove risky.

It is a good idea to start by enhancing the activities you already perform on a daily basis, building slowly to a more rigorous exercise regime. Here are some tips to start you off:

Try using the car less and think about all the trips you make that can be converted into walking events, rather than transported ones.

If you work in an environment that gives you a choice of stairs or using an elevator, use the stairs more to build up your aerobic capacity.

Play more with your kids, as vigorous episodes of playing outdoors is very beneficial regarding using opportunities for a good work out.

Take a moderately long walk after eating to aid digestion and work off those calories.

It is estimated that adults need about 2.5 hours of exercise each week, including activity that stretches the muscles. This is best maintained by spreading it out over the days, e.g. 30 minutes per day. People who are over the age of 65 probably have the capability to do just as much, but they may need to moderate the nature of the tasks and reduce the intensity of their exercise routine.

Ensure you have a good nights sleep

If you are unsure whether you sleep deeply or not, take another look at the section 'poor sleep patterns' and decide whether you can relate to some of the symptoms. Many of us know how frustrating it can trying to sleep through a partners snoring episode and the snorer and the frustrated partner may need to check this out with a health care professional, or access the advice of a sleep treatment clinic.

Sleeping after a day when you have taken the right amount of exercise is a whole lot easier than after a night watching TV on the couch.

When in doubt, check it out

If after reading this you feel that you are unsure about whether you are at more risk of contracting diabetes than you previously thought, then make sure you check out your concerns with a health care professional.

We cannot ever be 100% sure if issues like our ethnicity will ever impact upon our capacity to contract any disease, so if you are in doubt check it out.

If you are regularly taking steroids or any other medication – prescribed and non-prescribed, always check with your health care provider what the side effects are and if the prescriber has considered these risks in relation to other mitigating circumstances such as your family history, ethnicity and the effects of mixing medication with other prescribed medicine.

Smoking is now regarded as almost taboo now, and everyone should be aware of the inherent health risks. If you struggle to give up, once again, there are always plenty of health professionals or specialized alternative theorists who can help you.

5.
Conclusion

As we have seen, there is a personal responsibility attached to looking after our health.

A good place to start is arranging to visit your health care provider, and talk about your medical history, in an attempt to discover what risks are more likely to threaten your health. There are often things that we need to be aware of that we are not, and in the case of insulin resistance and Type 2 diabetes, we could be walking around like a human time bomb waiting to go off.

Take a look at your diet, the amount of exercise you take on a daily basis, how you sleep, what chemicals – this includes every prescribed and non-prescribed drug – and your ethnicity and then ask yourself if you think you may be at risk of a heightened chance of contracting insulin resistance, or Type 2 diabetes.

If you feel able to make the small adjustments you need to lessen the risks, then start work on them straight away. If you are unsure about how to make these changes, then ask your health care provider.

It is always going to be prudent to eat well, exercise regularly and ensure that you are aware of side effects relating to any drugs you ingest, therefore, carry out a stock take record and lessen your chances of becoming vulnerable to insulin resistance and Type 2 diabetes.

Good luck and remember, you only have one body and once it is worn out you cannot buy another one. Take this opportunity to become aware of the dangers of insulin resistance and Type 2 diabetes.

6. BONUSES!! FREE Stuff For You!

If You Want Free Best Selling Kindle Books Delivered to Your Inbox on a Weekly Basis

Head over to http://liveyourdreams.guru/free-kindle-book-club/

As a way of saying thank you for your purchase I am giving you an additional report FREE!! You can download this free report now! Simply head over to http://liveyourdreams.guru/diabetes-solution/

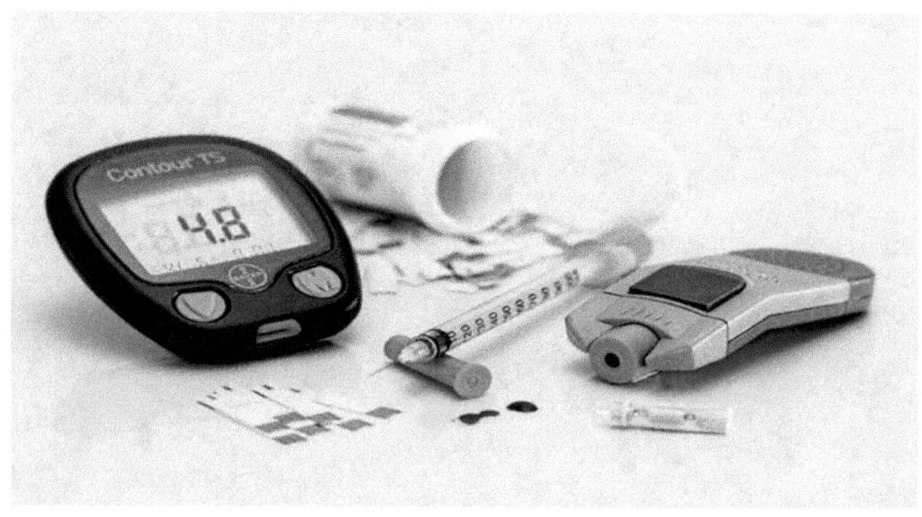